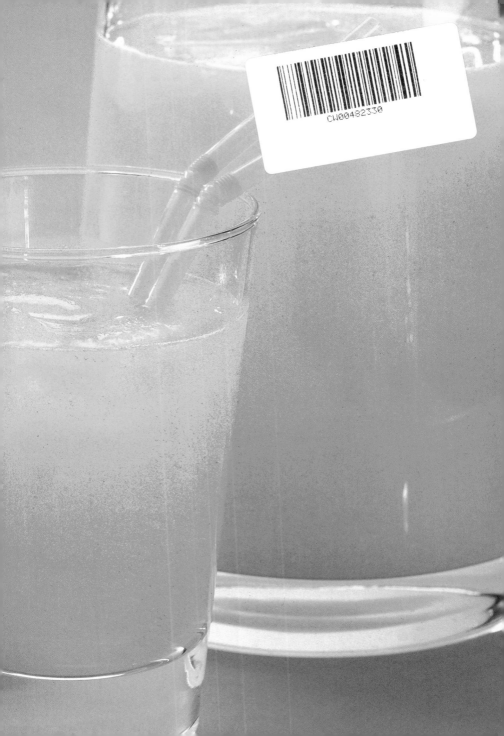

CW00482330

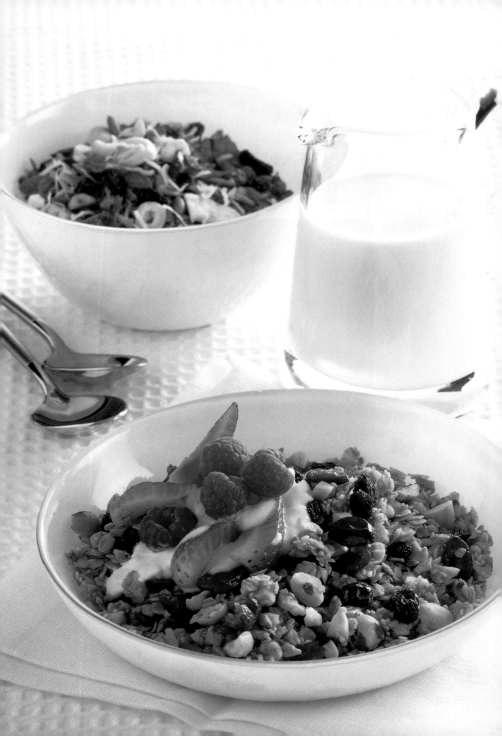

# 50 INSTANT WAYS TO
# ENERGIZE

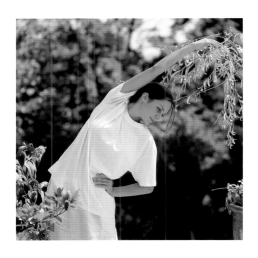

Practical ways to restore your
health and vibrancy

Tracey Kelly

LORENZ BOOKS

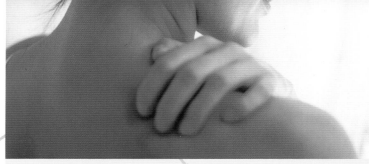

# contents

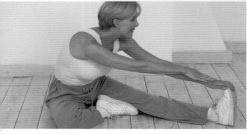

# 50 instant ways to

# energize

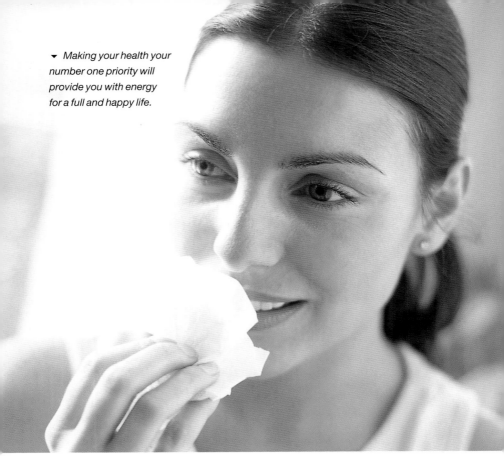

▾ *Making your health your number one priority will provide you with energy for a full and happy life.*

# introduction

As the pace of life in the 21st century becomes ever faster, some of us are left wondering, "Where will I ever find the energy to do all the things I need to do? Will I ever have some time left over for myself?"

The demands of partners, family, career, study, health and leisure pursuits seem to scream for constant attention. Whenever you are feeling frazzled and exhausted, bear in mind that you cannot do everything, and you can choose those people and things that are important to you. By making sure that you take care of yourself, you will ensure that you have the energy levels to deal with situations, happily and effectively.

This book sets out to help you uncover the great reserves of energy available to you, both physical and mental. By learning to pace yourself, you can accomplish all of your tasks — and still find time for yourself.

## taking stock

It can be a real revelation to take a day off to sort out your priorities: this alone will have a restorative effect on your vitality. The mind can easily go into overdrive, leaving you going around in circles and achieving nothing productive; taking steps to review your current expenditure of energy can help you "spend" it in more positive, efficient ways.

Maybe you've been grabbing junk food on the go, and perhaps you just haven't found the time to go swimming or play that game of squash in weeks. Could your insomnia be due to the huge amount of caffeine you've consumed to get you through the day? Maybe you've been feeling overwhelmed by the apparent seriousness of your life and its lack of enjoyment and fun.

You have a vague notion that your sluggish, lethargic feelings may be connected to these points, but you are unsure of what steps to take to correct the imbalances that harmful stimulants may have caused in the past.

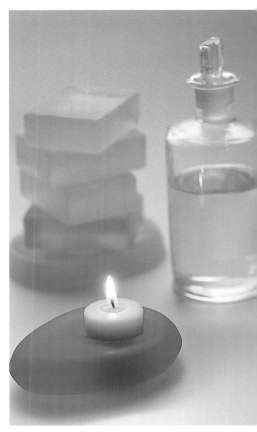

▲ *Take time out to pamper yourself with invigorating bath oils and fragrances.*

## energizing nutrition

It has often been said that "you are what you eat", and recent medical research has proved the validity of this old adage. Keeping a close watch on your daily diet – eating from a variety of fresh, unprocessed organic foods; staying hydrated by drinking plenty of water and low–caffeine herbal teas; keeping alcohol consumption at a moderate level – will ensure that you stay fit and alert. In particular, choosing foods that provide a good supply of the antioxidants – vitamins A, C and E – will help protect you from harmful pollution and chemicals in the environment, and waylay the onset of degenerative diseases.

## rejuvenating exercise

Many people are surprised when they discover that physical activity actually gives them more energy, not less. Exercise oxygenates the bloodstream and boosts the metabolism, providing a lasting stream of energy. And the long-term benefits of regular exercise are well-documented: it tones the muscles and works the heart, giving you a fighting chance for a fitter body as you grow older. By releasing substances called endorphins, it also helps to elevate your mood, leaving you in a brighter, more positive frame of mind that prepares you to face daily challenges with greater ease.

For maximum health value, it is best to include both aerobic and anaerobic exercises. Aerobic exercises are those that raise the pulse, burn fat, boost the immune system and exercise the heart, helping to prevent the build-up of arterial deposits that can lead to heart disease, one of the major killers. Walking, swimming, tennis, cycling and ball games provide a good workout and are enjoyable.

Anaerobics strengthen and tone the muscles, and build bone density, keeping at bay degenerative illnesses such as osteoporosis and back and joint problems. Examples include exercises where the muscles work at high intensity for short periods of time, such as weight lifting, squash and circuit training.

### powerful therapies

The healing powers of alternative therapies provide ways to work through physical and mental problems, and many are meditative and relaxing. Their effectiveness increases with regular use. Tactile therapies such as massage and reflexology work by manipulating muscles and pressure points to ease pain and discomfort. Colour and crystal healing use the energies of subtle vibrations to enliven and protect. With aromatherapy, the potent, active essences of plants and herbs are inhaled or absorbed through the skin – and their scent alone provides a delightful mood lift.

### sensual pampering

It is important not to forget that feeling attractive is an essential part of your energizing plan. Pampering your body with the delicious fragrances and textures of some of the spa treatments included in this book will help you to look and feel your best. Invigorating body scrubs and bath oils cleanse and hydrate the skin, and homemade hair rinses and skin fresheners prepare you to face the world with renewed grace and beauty.

### lighten your load

Contrary to popular belief, taking regular breaks from normal activity actually increases your productivity, whether at work, at home or in dealing with family matters. Especially when under stress, taking time out to "recharge the batteries" can be a life-saver. It is easy to carry out self-help practices, from deep breathing techniques to taking a walk around the block – often, it is simply a matter of remembering to do so. Enjoyable activities such as dancing and having a laugh enliven your spirits, giving you the motivation to perform all the practical tasks you have to accomplish.

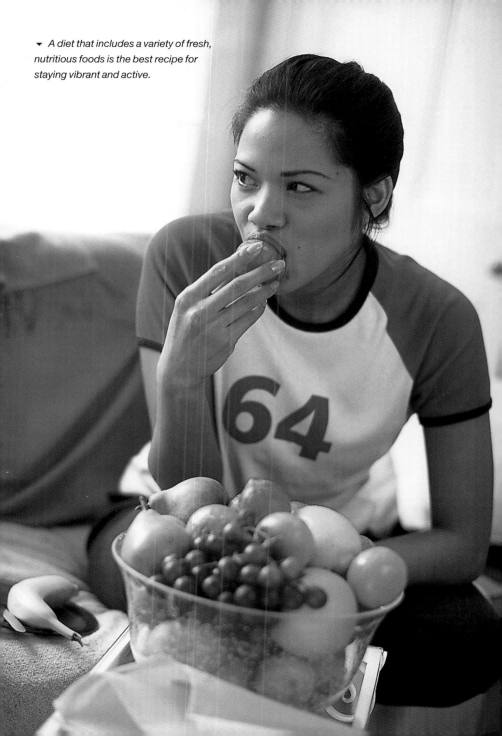

A diet that includes a variety of fresh, nutritious foods is the best recipe for staying vibrant and active.

# energizing
# treatments

Increase your vitality by choosing from the following ideas for fighting fatigue and giving yourself an energizing boost, whether short or longer term. A selection of revitalizing foods, drinks, vitamins, exercises, beauty treatments and therapies will help set you on the road to a fit and healthy body and a lively, productive mind.

Diet is an important part of an active lifestyle, and it is essential that you get enough nutrients from food. Here you will find information on the health-giving properties of meat, fish and poultry; fruits and vegetables; grains, nuts and pulses. You'll also find recipes for delicious juices, tisanes and shakes.

Aerobic, t'ai chi and yoga exercises are all satisfying ways to increase your physical stamina. Also included are reflexology, aromatherapy and crystal healing therapies, which improve the body's flow of energy. Instant energy fixes such as clearing your mind will remind you that you have the power to make your life as fulfilling and exciting as it can be.

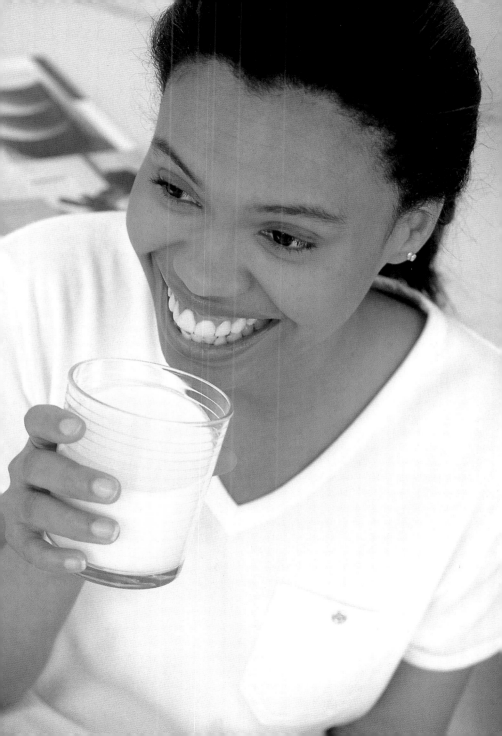

# 1

# vital vitamin C

This important energizing vitamin is essential for maintaining a healthy and resilient immune system. Vitamin C helps the body absorb iron from vegetable sources. It also helps fight off colds and flu.

Also known as ascorbic acid, vitamin C assists with tissue growth, the healing of wounds, and the prevention of blood clotting and bruising. It is a powerful antioxidant, which – when taken with vitamins A and E – helps curtail the effects of pollution on the body. A shortage of vitamin C can result in water retention, a lack of energy, poor digestion, colds and bronchial infections. Some good food sources of vitamin C include berries, citrus fruits, green leafy vegetables, guavas, tomatoes, melons and peppers.

## cooking care

Vitamin C is particularly unstable and is easily destroyed by heat, so it is a good idea to get your intake by eating plenty of fresh, raw fruits and vegetables. It is best to buy organic produce, and prepare just before eating to preserve as much of the vitamin content as possible. Keep a well-stocked fruit bowl for a quick energy boost between meals.

▶ *Oranges and lemons provide the body with a very accessible form of vitamin C.*

**SUPPLEMENTS**
As a supplement, vitamin C is more effective if it is taken along with bioflavonoids, calcium and magnesium (it aids calcium absorption). The RDA is only 60mg, but many health practitioners recommend higher doses to keep disease at bay – somewhere between 200-500mg for healthy adults. If you feel you need more vitamin C, consult your doctor before taking larger amounts.

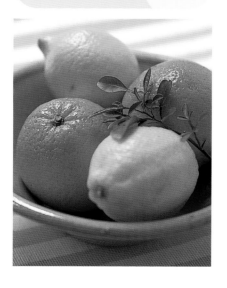

# 2

# rejuvenating vitamin E

An essential fat-soluble substance, vitamin E helps increase stamina and endurance and, not only does it promote fertility, it is reported to spice up your sex life as well.

Vitamin E contains several antioxidant compounds that help the body fight free radicals, to which we all are vulnerable via pollution and food additives. Vitamin E is also known to prevent degenerative diseases such as heart disease, arthritis, diabetes and cancer. Plenty of vitamin E keeps your skin looking younger and glowing, and actually helps keep wrinkles at bay. Vitamin E oil can be used on the skin as a soothing, topical treatment for eczema, cold sores, skin ulcers and shingles. A deficiency in vitamin E is not very common, but signs may include fatigue, premature aging, inflamed varicose or thread veins, and wounds that are slow to heal.

## how to get it

Vitamin E is found in many types of foods, including nuts, seeds such as sunflower and pumpkin, cold-pressed oils, vegetables, spinach, whole grains, wheatgerm oil, asparagus, avocado, beef, seafood, apples, carrots and celery. As a food supplement, vitamin E is best taken with other antioxidants – vitamin C, betacarotene (vitamin A) and selenium; an element important in maintaining a healthy immune system and enhancing a positive frame of mind. The RDA for women is 8mg and around 10mg for men.

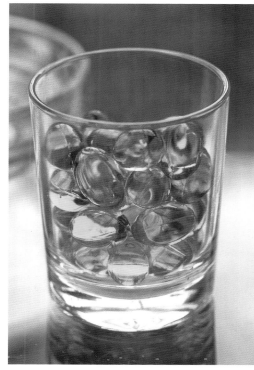

▲ Vitamin E supplements come in different strengths – choose a low dose to start with.

# 3 B-complex vitamins

The B group vitamins are vital for their role in releasing energy from food, providing the body with a steady stream of nutrients. Eat a variety of B-rich foods, as they work in tandem with each other.

The best way to get B vitamins is from natural food sources, although there are many good-quality B-complex supplements available. Vegetarians in particular may need to top up their $B_{12}$ intake by using a supplement. Care should be taken, as a sensitivity to niacin may result in a temporary rash or headache for 15–30 minutes. The B vitamins are better taken in the early part of the day, as they provide a real physical and mental boost.

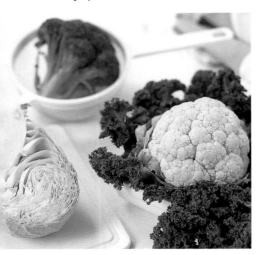

▲ Like vitamin C, Bs are water soluble and easily destroyed – take care when cooking.

**CRUCIAL B VITAMINS**

• Vitamin $B_1$ (thiamin): Enhances circulation; boosts brain power. Foods: seeds, beans, peanuts, bran, liver, pork, seafood, egg-yolk.

• Vitamin $B_2$ (riboflavin): Helps metabolize amino acids, fatty acids and carbohydrates. Foods: nuts, eggs, dairy, vegetables, meats.

• Vitamin $B_3$ (niacin): Promotes circulation, healthy skin and nerves. Foods: liver, poultry, fish, rabbit, nuts, yeast, cereals, legumes.

• Vitamin $B_5$ (pantothenic acid): Aids hormone secretion; helps fight allergies. Foods: beef, eggs, fish, kidney, legumes, mushrooms.

• Vitamin $B_6$ (pyridoxine): Helps balance female hormones and fight depression. Foods: chicken, fish, liver, kidney, eggs, walnuts, carrots.

• Vitamin $B_9$: Aids red blood cell formation. Foods: spinach, beans, broccoli, vegetables, whole grains.

• Vitamin $B_{12}$ (cyanocobamin): Helps sharpen mental processes. Foods: liver, red meat, shellfish, eggs, cheese, fish.

# 4 essential minerals

Energizing minerals such as magnesium, zinc and iron play a vital role in regulating the body's functions. They are constituents of all body tissues and fluids, and work to stimulate the immune system.

## invigorating magnesium

Take plenty of magnesium to boost energy levels – a deficiency can lead to tiredness and irritability. It helps the body absorb calcium, so it is important for the formation of bone and teeth, and also helps control blood pressure. To consume enough of the mineral, choose from a wide selection of magnesium-rich foods, including dairy products, fish, meat, legumes, apples, apricots, avocados, bananas, wholegrain cereals, nuts, dark green vegetables and cocoa.

## activating zinc

Especially important for the growth of muscle tissue and for maintaining a healthy and active immune system, zinc is often used with vitamin C to fight colds, sore throats and flu. Skin problems such as acne also benefit

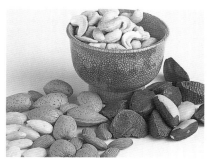

▲ Nuts are bursting with essential minerals such as zinc, magnesium and selenium.

from zinc, and a good supply will keep hair, skin and nails healthy. To get enough zinc, eat plenty of meat, poultry, fish, nuts, eggs, seeds, whole grains and brewer's yeast.

## energizing iron

Essential in the production of red blood cells, iron is important for sustaining energy levels. Symptoms of deficiency include fatigue, muscular weakness, nervousness and shortness of breath. Include liver, meat, egg yolks, dark green leafy vegetables, legumes and nuts in your diet. Orange juice drunk with a vegetarian meal will help the body absorb iron.

> **CAUTION**
> Before taking any type of iron supplement, consult your doctor, as iron can be harmful in large doses. A fatal dose for children could be as little as 600mg.

# 5 vitalizing fruit & vegetables

Fruit and vegetables are storehouses of energizing nutrients. Packed with vitamins, minerals, fibre and enzymes, raw fruit and vegetables are the perfect snack, and are easy to eat at any time of day.

## refreshing fruit

Fruit such as apples, pears, mangoes, strawberries and grapes provide a steady stream of energy via fructose, a natural sugar. Apples also contain malic acid, which boosts digestion. Citrus fruits are packed with vitamin C, a powerful antioxidant that protects the body against harmful free radicals, inhibits premature aging and increases iron absorption. Freshly squeezed oranges and grapefruits stimulate the digestion and tone the whole system. They are also a good source of betacarotene, calcium, phosphorus and potassium.

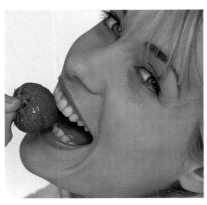

▲ Strawberries make an ideal quick snack.

## handy dried fruit

Higher in calories than fresh fruit, dried fruit provides plenty of sustaining energy for a busy day. Unlike other high-sugar foods, such as chocolate and sweets, dried fruit is an excellent source of nutrients. For an easily portable, fast energy snack, look for unsulphured fruit, such as dried hunza apricots, figs, dates, raisins, currants, apples and peaches.

## vitamin-rich vegetables

Known for their calming effect on the body, vegetables balance acid and alkaline levels and provide essential nutrients. A large salad at lunchtime will fill you up and is satisfyingly crunchy. Raw spinach is an excellent choice – it contains betacarotene (vitamin A), vitamin C, calcium, folate, iron, potassium, thiamin and zinc.

With a rich supply of vitamin A, carrots have the effect of stimulating the whole body. They are easy to clean and carry for a quick snack. Members of the cruciferous family – broccoli, cauliflower, cabbage, Brussels sprouts and watercress – stimulate the liver, and keep the digestive system active.

# 6 healthy whole grains

Whole grains and cereals are vital ingredients in a healthy, energizing diet. Not only are they an excellent source of low-fat protein, they contain carbohydrates, fibre, vitamins and minerals.

## bountiful grains

Grains have been a part of the human diet for thousands of years, and have been cultivated for centuries. To glean a variety of the best nutrients, include a selection of different grains in your diet, such as brown rice, barley, millet, oats, buckwheat and quinoa. A bowl of brown rice with lightly steamed vegetables will work to steady the nervous system.

For a breakfast with staying power, try a bowl of porridge – oats absorb impurities in the blood, leaving your skin glowing. For tasty variety, add a few chopped nuts, raisins or apricots. The South American grain, quinoa, contains more protein than any other – a good choice for times when you need to be on top form all day.

## essential fibre

Unprocessed whole grains contain soluble and insoluble fibre, both of which are fundamental in the prevention of constipation, colon and rectal cancers, ulcers and heart disease. Foods rich in fibre bind with harmful cholesterol and help it to pass through the body for elimination.

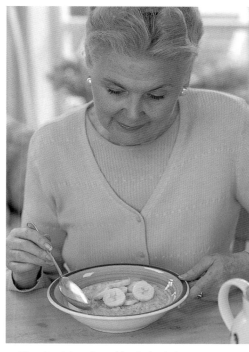

▲ *The starch in oat porridge helps to keep blood sugar levels on an even keel.*

Bread is a good source of fibre; aim to eat about six slices a day. Vary the types so that you include different grains, for example, alternate whole-wheat, rye, multigrain, oat and millet.

# 7 energy-sustaining pulses

Providing essential low-fat protein, fibre and vitamins, pulses have long been a staple of vegetarian diets. They are bursting with minerals – including folate, iron, magnesium and potassium.

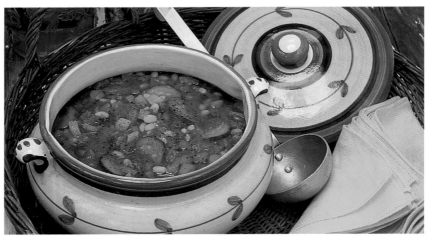

**large choice**

Pulses include beans and legumes such as lentils, dried peas, pinto and mung beans, chickpeas and soya beans. It is preferable to use dry beans in cooking, as processing often adds sugar and salt. For a nourishing and energy-giving lunch, try eating a stew or thick soup made from a selection of tasty beans and vegetables. Alternatively, try delicious baked dishes based on butter (lima) or pinto beans.

Most dried beans need to be soaked for at least eight hours before cooking. Leave overnight in a covered

▲ *Bean soups provide a steady energy flow through the slow release of carbohydrates.*

pan with plenty of cold water. The next morning, drain and rinse before boiling hard for at least 10 minutes, then leave them to simmer until cooked. Alternatively, follow your recipe for cooking instructions.

**bean sensitivity**

Never eat beans raw or partially cooked; they may cause an allergic reaction. When trying a new type of bean, eat a small amount first to test.

# 8 brain-boosting fish

Fish is often called "brain food" as it is high in protein, B vitamins, minerals and Omega fatty acids. It is best to include several varieties as part of your energizing diet.

White fish is a good choice as it is very low in fat. Oily fish – such as sardines, mackerel, herring, tuna, trout and salmon – provide large amounts of vitamins A and D. They also provide Omega fatty acids, which are beneficial in helping to prevent coronary heart diseases, and leave the skin looking fresh and clear.

## choice cooking methods
There are a number of fast and delicious ways to cook fish. Almost any cooking method suits fish except boiling, although simmering is fine for healthy soups.

Since fish is so delicate, it is better to undercook than overcook it. Because of many factors – the variety, weight and thickness of the flesh – it is impossible to give exact cooking times for a portion of fish, but it is considered cooked when the internal temperature has reached 63°C/145°F.

Fish can be baked, braised, fried, stir-fried, grilled (broiled), barbecued, microwaved and seared. To test whether fish fillets are done, part the flesh with a small knife; the flesh should look opaque rather than translucent. Next, gently ease the flesh off the bone; it should come away but not fall off easily.

## cold preparation
Very fresh fish may be prepared without heat by being marinated or soused with lemon juice or flavoured vinegar – the acids soften the flesh and turn it opaque. One classic dish that uses this method is ceviche, where cubes or strips of firm white fish, such as halibut, cod, snapper and turbot, are marinated in lemon juice, salt and chopped chillis for two hours. Japanese sushi uses very fresh fish often rolled in seaweed, and garnished with vinegar and wasabi, a very hot mustard.

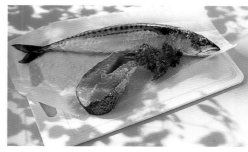

▲ Fish is an ideal food – it is a delicious source of protein and important nutrients.

# 9 wholesome eggs

Eggs contain the most complete nutrition of any food – all encased in a tidy package with a long shelf-life. They provide energy-boosting protein, iron, zinc and vitamins A, E and B complex.

## a good egg

Easily accessible and inexpensive, eggs can be a wonderful addition to a healthy and energizing diet. When eaten in moderation, there is no need to fear excessive intake of cholesterol. Made up of white (albumen) and yolk, an egg consists of water, fat and protein, with smaller amounts of other essential nutrients and minerals. The white contains water and protein, while the yolk contains fat, protein and vitamins. To take advantage of their complete nutrition, eggs should be enjoyed whole; organic, free-range (farm-fresh) varieties of chicken and duck eggs offer the best quality and taste.

## the perfect ingredient

Eggs are easy to cook and incredibly versatile, lending themselves to many exciting dishes such as omelettes, quiches, frittatas, custards and soufflés. They also provide a quick and delicious meal on their own, following one of many cooking methods: they can be hard- or soft-boiled, fried, scrambled, poached or baked.

Controlling the heat and cooking time are the keys to preparing eggs successfully. Generally, when making plain cooked eggs, the temperature should not be too high – they can easily burn, as in frying; or they may lose taste and texture when over-boiled, poached or baked.

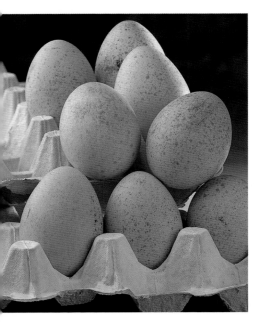

◄ *With so many egg dishes to choose from – both sweet and savoury – you're bound to find an energizing recipe to suit your tastes.*

# 10 protein-packed poultry

A good source of quality protein, B vitamins and some iron, poultry is also low in fat if the skin is removed. Preferably choose organic, free-range poultry to ensure it is healthy and nutritious.

### light meal, anytime

Ideal for use in an energizing diet, high-protein chicken and other poultry such as turkey, duck and guinea fowl offer many benefits in terms of nutrition and taste. Poultry is extremely versatile and complements many side dishes: vegetables, potatoes, grains such as rice and couscous, and even fruit – it is delicious prepared with tangy apricots and cranberries.

### preparing poultry

Poultry may be used whole or cut into pieces for cooking. It can be prepared using a variety of methods, from grilling (broiling), baking and frying, to barbecuing, roasting and boiling; or it can be added to a variety of casseroles, soups and stir-fries.

It is essential to arrive at the right cooking time and temperature: poultry must never be eaten undercooked, as bacteria may be lurking; and if overcooked, the meat will be tough and stringy.

To make roast chicken – one of the easiest and most delicious poultry dishes – use the following guidelines: preheat the oven to 200°C/400°F/Gas 6.

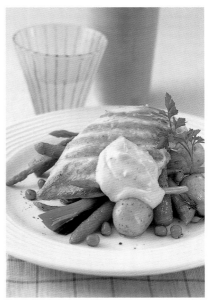

▲ *Escalopes of chicken are quick and easy to prepare – they are simple, tasty and highly nutritious.*

Weigh the bird after it has been trimmed and stuffed, and place in a roasting pan in the hot oven. Allow 20 minutes of cooking time per 450g/1lb, plus an extra 20 minutes. With a very large bird, cover with foil until the final 15 minutes of cooking.

# 11 iron-rich meat & game

Although the general health advice is to moderate your intake of red meat, thus reducing saturated fat, it is still the best source of readily absorbed iron, zinc and B vitamins – all crucial for boosting energy.

Today's meat is leaner than formerly, and if low-fat cooking methods are used, it can fit into the profile of a healthy diet and provide you with plenty of sustained energy. Choose organic lamb, beef and pork, and free-range game to ensure that the meat is safe, free from hormones and additives, and comes from farms where animal welfare is a priority.

Pan frying is probably the most traditional way of cooking beef or game sirloins, fillets and chops. Start by taking a heavy pan, preferably non-stick, and rub it with just a light coating of sunflower or safflower oil. Heat the pan and add a knob (pat) of butter, which should melt immediately.

Trim excess fat from the steak or chop, and cook following the times given below. Use a draining spoon or fish slice (metal spatula) to transfer the steak to the plate. You can then serve with a selection of side dishes, such as rice or potatoes, roasted or stir-fried vegetables and green salads.

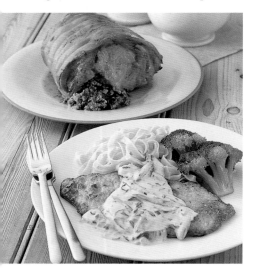

### cooking times for red meat
*For very rare steak*: cut about 2.5cm/1in thick and allow 1 minute for each side for fillet; for rump (round steak), allow 2 minutes per side.
*For rare steak*: allow 2 minutes each side for fillet; 3 minutes for rump.
*For medium rare steak*: allow 2-3 minutes for each side for fillet; 2-4 minutes for rump.
*For well-done steak*: allow 3 minutes each side, then reduce heat and allow a further 5–10 minutes.

◀ *Include meat in your diet to supply your body with a full range of nutrients.*

# 12

# essential fats & oils

Choosing the right fat is vital for sustaining energy levels and overall health. Plant oils provide essential fatty acids and vitamin E, beneficial for heart and skin. Animal fats should be used in moderation.

While butter and cream may be eaten occasionally, plant oils offer a healthier option for supplying essential energizing nutrients found in fats. High in unsaturated fats, olive, sunflower, safflower and grapeseed oils are all good choices to include in your daily diet. Speciality oils such as walnut, sesame, almond and hazelnut are a tasty alternative. Some of the essential substances in oils are lost during heated processing, so look for organic, cold-pressed oils, which retain most of their nutritional value.

### mediterranean olive dressing

250ml/8fl oz/1 cup olive oil
120ml/4fl oz/½ cup freshly squeezed
    lemon juice
50ml/2fl oz/¼ cup water
10ml/2 tsps brown sugar
2.5ml/½ tsp each of oregano, thyme,
    sage and marjoram
salt and freshly ground black pepper

Place oil, lemon juice and water in a bottle. Add the herbs, then a dash of salt and black pepper. Shake well and add the dressing to salads or use as a marinade for roast vegetables.

▼ *The delicate flavour of sunflower oil will not overpower any dish.*

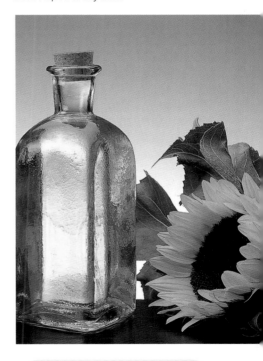

Almond oil is an excellent choice for a revitalizing massage, as it is easily absorbed into the skin.

# 13 nutritious nuts & seeds

Protein-rich nuts and seeds give a more sustained energy boost than carbohydrates, and are a good alternative to meat. The vitamin E content of nuts also helps the condition of skin, hair and nails.

Nuts contain essential nutrients, such as B vitamins, calcium, iron, potassium, magnesium, phosphorus and essential fatty acids. They also contain selenium – just three brazil nuts provide the daily requirement.

**versatile nuts**
Walnuts, almonds, cashews, hazelnuts, brazil nuts and peanuts offer some of the best health benefits – they can be eaten on their own, or added to porridge, breads, casseroles and salads. Since they have a high oil content (albeit unsaturated), keep in mind that nuts are high in calories and should be eaten in moderation.

**nutritious seeds**
Seeds such as pumpkin, sunflower and sesame offer similar nutritional values with slightly fewer calories. Buy them in small quantities, seal and store in a cool place. Wholegrain toast spread with tahini (crushed sesame seed spread) or peanut butter makes a nutritious start to the day, and will provide energy all morning.

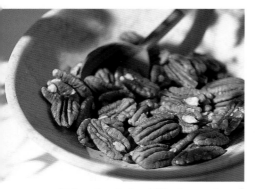

▲ *Nuts make a tasty addition to cereals and porridge. You can also add them to stir-fries, breads, cakes and biscuits (cookies).*

▶ *For sustained energy, eat a handful of nuts before exercising, or take some along while outdoors on a long hike.*

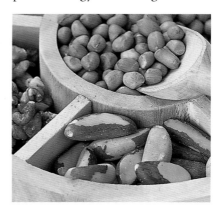

# 14 cleansing garlic

Containing antiviral and antibacterial nutrients, garlic acts to cleanse and energize the immune system. It is said to protect against disease and bacteria, lower cholesterol levels and fight cancer.

The plant's historical use has been documented for 5,000 years. Often called nature's strongest antibiotic, it was used to prevent the plague in France in the early 1700s, and in the trenches to fight gangrene in World Wars I and II. Garlic is reputed to bestow all kinds of health benefits, from increasing overall physical strength and vitality, to reducing lethargy – so if you're feeling "under the weather" generally, a good place to start energizing may be to up your intake of garlic.

### tasty addition

Add fresh garlic to olive or walnut oil for a piquant salad dressing. It is also delicious cooked in main dishes such as stir-fries, casseroles and soups. If you do not like the taste or smell of garlic, try taking deodorized garlic supplements, which are available from health food shops and chemists.

### garlic bread

Another delicious way to boost your intake is to make garlic bread as part of a lunch or dinner menu. Crush two bulbs of garlic and infuse in

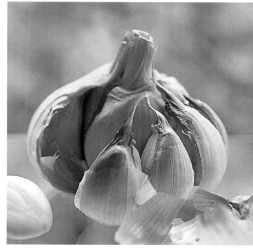

▲ Garlic is one of the most renowned "miracle cures" in nearly all cultures. It is added to many dishes – even desserts!

120ml/4 fl oz/½ cup of olive oil an hour previous to serving time. Take slices of wholemeal (whole-wheat), rye, mixed grain or white bread, and brush each side with the garlic oil. Heat until slightly crisp in a preheated oven (160°C/325°F/Gas 3) for 10–15 minutes, depending on the thickness of the slices. Serve warm with pasta or a ragout of vegetables.

# hydrating water

Water is an essential nutrient that is vital for bodily functions and sustaining activity levels. It is lost constantly through sweat, urination and exhaling vapour, and must be replenished regularly.

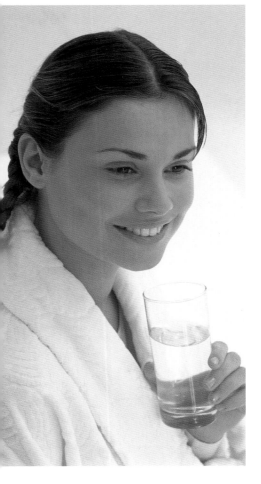

### healthy hydration

Pure mineral or filtered tap water will flush toxins from your organs, leaving you feeling rejuvenated and your skin glowing and healthy. Diluted fruit and vegetable juices are also good choices. Avoid soft drinks that contain sugar, preservatives and flavourings – they will give you a temporary "sugar" high, but you will feel tired an hour later when the effect wears off. Carbonated water is acceptable, drunk in small amounts, but try to find low-sodium brands.

### top up your intake

It is a good idea to drink a large and refreshing glass of still water when you wake in the morning, as your body dehydrates during the night, especially in warm or hot weather. Do not rely on your sense of thirst to tell you when to drink: keep sipping throughout the day. A glass of cold water is refreshing and has a restorative effect on the senses.

◄ *The best way to keep hydrated is to drink up to 2 litres/3½ pints/8½ cups daily – more if it is hot outside or you are exercising heavily.*

# 16 fruit & vegetable juices

Fresh fruit and vegetable juices are an ideal way to give yourself an energy boost. They stimulate the system, providing fructose – a slow-burning sugar – and plentiful vitamins and minerals.

## cranberry and apple juice

This refreshing juice boosts the metabolism first thing in the morning.

4 eating apples
600ml/1 pint/2½ cups cranberry juice
2.5cm/1 in fresh root ginger,
    peeled and grated

Peel the apples, if you wish, then core and chop them. Pour the cranberry juice into the food processor or blender, then add the apples and ginger and process for a few minutes until smooth. Serve chilled.

## zingy vegetable juice

The ginger in this juice packs a powerful punch, giving you a lift in the afternoon.

1 beetroot (beet), cooked in its
    natural juice
1 large carrot, sliced
4cm/1½ in piece fresh root ginger,
    peeled and grated
2 apples, peeled, cored and chopped
150g/5oz/1¼ cups seedless
    white grapes
300ml/½ pints fresh orange juice

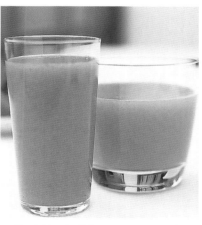

▲ Fresh blended juices are easy to make.

Place the beetroot, carrot, ginger, apples, grapes and orange juice in a food processor or blender and process for a few minutes until smooth. Serve immediately, or chill and serve later.

### JUICING TIPS
• Juices speed up the metabolism and improve energy levels.
• Drink fruit juices with breakfast – their sugars kick-start the system.
• Vegetable juices are best drunk in the afternoon, as they re-establish the body's acid and alkaline balance.

Herbal teas hydrate and refresh the body without straining the cardio-vascular system. Mint tea is especially stimulating when energy levels are low.

# 18 fragrant tisanes

Tisanes are teas made by seeping sprigs of garden-fresh leaves and flowers in boiling water. They provide a treat for the senses, and can give you an instant physical and psychological boost.

The experience of drinking tisanes is a little bit like taking the garden's growing energy into your body. The wonderful fragrances of these clean and clear tonics act as mood enhancers, and they provide a visual treat – as well as tasting wonderfully fresh. Many blossoms can be used for making tisanes, such as dandelion, rosemary, rose petals, lavender, lime blossom, peppermint, lemon verbena, jasmine and bergamot.

### rosemary tisane

This familiar garden plant contains several active, aromatic oils. The action of rosemary is such that it stimulates as it increases the blood supply to the brain, keeping the mind clear and aiding concentration. Rosemary will also relieve nervous tension and combat fatigue. It is ideal from a culinary point of view, in that it is a sturdy evergreen shrub, from which leaf sprigs can be cut all year round.

To make a tea, place one sprig of rosemary (or 10ml/2 tsp dried herb) in a cup and add 250ml/8fl oz/ 1 cup boiling water. Infuse for 4 minutes before removing the sprig.

▾ *A wonderful way to revive tired senses, tisanes are tasty and aromatic.*

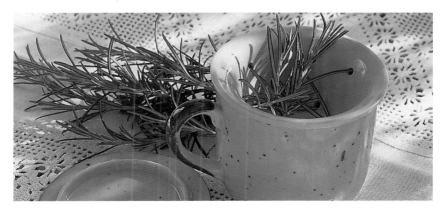

# 19  fruit shakes

More nutritious than the fat- and calorie-laden ice-cream variety, fresh fruit shakes supply an immediate and lasting burst of fructose, providing you with sustained energy for hours.

## mixed berry yogurt shake

250ml/8fl oz/1 cup semi-skimmed milk, chilled
250ml/8fl oz/1 cup low-fat natural yogurt
115g/4oz mixed berries
5ml/1 tsp rosewater
a little honey, to taste

Blend the milk, yogurt, fruits and rosewater in a food processor, and process until frothy. Add honey to taste; this will depend on the sweetness of the fruits. Pour into tall glasses and serve.

## citrus shake

1 pineapple
6 oranges, peeled and chopped
1 lemon, juiced
1 pink grapefruit, peeled and chopped

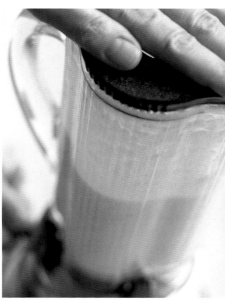

▲ The vitamin C and mineral content of fruit shakes provides much of the RDA – and they are wonderfully tasty, too!

Prepare the pineapple by cutting the bottom and spiky top off the fruit. Stand upright and cut off the skin, removing all the spikes and as little of the flesh as possible.

Lay the pineapple on its side and cut into bite-size chunks. Place the pineapple, oranges, lemon juice and grapefruit in a food processor or blender, and process for a few minutes until the ingredients are combined. Press the fruit juice through a sieve to remove any pith or membranes. Serve chilled with breakfast or a snack.

# 20 fruit smoothies

A combination of soft-textured fruits and yogurt, smoothies are easy to make and offer a tasty alternative to eating plain fruit as part of an energy-boosting eating plan.

### banana and strawberry smoothie

Packed with energy–giving oats and fruit, this smoothie makes a perfect start to the day.

2 bananas, quartered
250g/9oz strawberries
30ml/2 tbsp oatmeal
550ml/18fl oz/2½ cups natural
    live yogurt

Peel and chop the banana into large chunks; top the strawberries. Place the ingredients in a food processor or blender and process until creamy. Pour the smoothie mixture into tall glasses and serve.

### plum and mango smoothie

150g/5oz fresh plums
300g/11oz mango
15ml/1 tbsp honey
550ml/18fl oz/2½ cups natural
    live yogurt

Stone (pit) the plums, peel and chop the mango into large chunks. Place the ingredients in a food processor or blender. Process for 1-2 minutes until frothy. Pour into large glasses and serve.

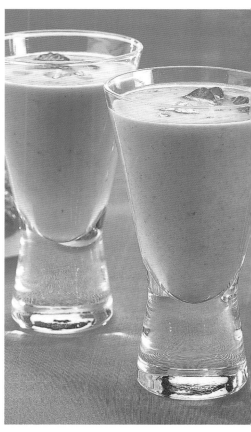

▲ *Experiment with combinations of your favourite fruits. For maximum nutritional content, serve smoothies immediately.*

# 21 aerobic exercise

Sustained by oxygen, aerobic exercises raise the heart rate for prolonged periods. They burn fat, boost the immune system and leave you with an energy surplus that increases general stamina.

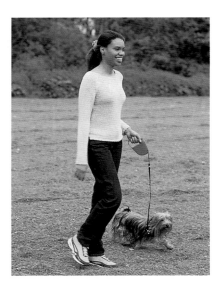

*◀ Aerobic exercise helps to increase and stabilize your stamina and energy levels.*

could alternate swimming with tennis. Remember to drink plenty of water when you exercise, as you can easily become dehydrated.

**endless choice**
Tennis, badminton, walking, jogging, cycling and swimming all offer excellent aerobic exercise – with the bonus being that they are inexpensive and enjoyable. Most gyms offer classes that use steps or weights, and some have tennis and badminton courts. Many offer dance classes in diverse styles as well. Choose an activity that matches your fitness level.

**extra stamina**
Aerobics will help give a real boost to your stamina and overall fitness levels. If you are feeling tired or frustrated, go for a walk or do some simple exercises for 10-15 minutes – note how energized you feel afterwards.

You should aim to do your chosen aerobics exercise for 45 minutes, three times a week, and it is a good idea to vary what you do, so that you don't become bored. For example, you

**AEROBIC TIPS**
• Choose an exercise that you enjoy: if you find the gym boring, try dancing, tennis or walking.
• Once you get started, the benefits will be such that you won't want to stop. Your mental outlook will improve as well: exercise helps to keep depression at bay.

# 22 anaerobic exercise

An exercise made up of short bursts of activity is called anaerobic. The muscles work intensely for short periods and, with continued exercise, they become stronger, providing you with more energy.

## building strength

Muscle tissue is lost as the body ages, so it is important to begin building a strong physique as early as possible. And with physical strength comes confidence – a precious attribute that will see you through all of life's uncertainties. Strive to create an exercise regime that works for you, one that you can incorporate easily and enjoyably into your daily routine.

You can ask for advice on anaerobics at your local gym: many of the instructors are trained to offer an initial consultation on workouts and diet. Personal trainers offer a programme that is tailored to your own changing needs.

## fighting fit

Before beginning a new anaerobics regime, check with your doctor if you have back or joint problems. Always do warm-up stretches, especially before using weights or playing squash, as cold muscles and ligaments can easily become strained.

Anaerobics result in the build-up of lactic acid in the muscles, causing temporary discomfort, which is why they cannot be sustained for long – lactic acid must leave the muscles before you can continue.

At the start of a new exercise, it is wise to limit yourself to 15-20 minutes a session, gradually increasing this as your strength increases. Always stop exercising if you are in pain.

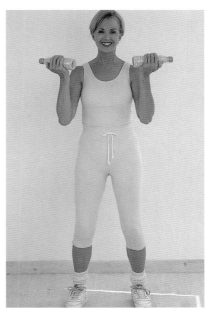

▲ *Anaerobic exercises help increase your energy levels by improving muscle mass.*

# 23 stimulating stretches

Chronic tension can easily lead to fatigue and exhaustion. When your memory and concentration suffer and stress leads to constant tiredness, these exercises may be helpful.

### shoulder stand

**1** Lie on your back, with your legs straight out and your arms by your side. Raise your legs until vertical. Continue lifting them over your head while raising your buttocks off the floor. **2** Supporting your lower back with your hands, slowly bring your back and legs to the vertical position. **3** Hold for a few moments, then return to the original position.

*Caution*: Avoid inverted position exercises if pregnant, and always seek medical advice if you suffer from high blood pressure or an overactive thyroid.

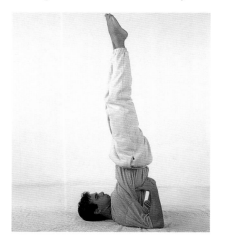

### fish posture

**1** Lie flat on your back. **2** Arch your back until the top of your head is resting on the floor. Hold the position, then relax.

*Caution*: This exercise is best avoided by those with neck problems.

### leg clasp

**1** Stand upright with your feet together. Bending forwards, clasp your hands behind your legs, as far down as is comfortable. **2** Steadily pull your head towards your legs. Go only as far as you can manage without strain. Hold for a few moments, then slowly uncurl and return to an upright position.

### backwards bend

**1** Stand with your hands on your hips, and your feet slightly apart. **2** Breathe in, then exhale as you bend backwards from the waist. Do not go further than is comfortable.

*Caution*: Avoid this stretch if you have any back problems.

◀ *Stretches bring blood to the brain and help boost your mental agility and mood.*

# 24 refreshing water sports

Sports that take place in or around water are, by their very nature, exhilarating. They range from the adventurous – sailing, water skiing, snorkelling, surfing and scuba diving – to healthy swimming.

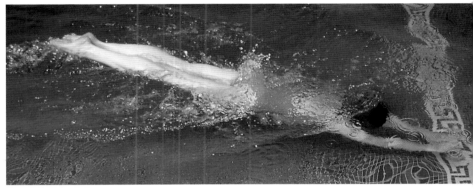

## stimulating swimming

One of the most complete exercises you can do, swimming works all of the major muscle groups of the body without putting strain on the joints and spine – so people of all levels of fitness can enjoy the activity.

An exercise that is both aerobic and anaerobic, vigorous swimming also burns up anywhere between 500-700 calories an hour – so if you're trying to lose weight while you energize, this is a good choice. It will also raise your metabolism for several hours afterwards, meaning that you will burn more calories even at rest. To make the most of the activity, it is best to brush up on your strokes

▲ *Simple swimming is a great exercise, available at most local leisure centres.*

and make sure you have the proper form. If you paddle with your head above the water, you may be placing strain on your neck and shoulders, exacerbating back pain.

## everyone in the water

It can be fun and invigorating to share exercise with a group. Classes in water aerobics, swimming and yoga are held at most pools, and some offer scuba diving as well. While on holiday, why not try snorkelling, or lessons in water skiing, sailing and surfing, all of which are challenging and rewarding.

# 25

## energy-channelling t'ai chi

Practised by millions of Chinese, T'ai Chi Chuan combines exercise with meditation. Its emphasis is on channelling and helping the flow of energy, or "chi", rather than simply building physical strength.

**cloud hands**

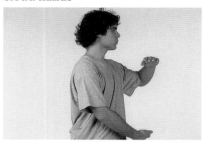

**1** Begin with your right hand facing your navel, your left hand directly above it, facing your chest. Slowly turn your waist to the left, shifting your weight on to your left leg. At the same time, turn your palms towards each other, as if holding a large ball.

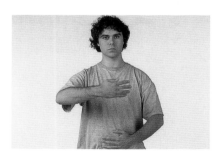

**2** Bring your waist back to the front. As you do so, lower your left hand until it is opposite the navel and raise your right hand to the level of your chest, with your palms facing your body.

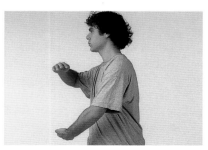

**3** Now turn your waist to the right, shifting the weight across to your right leg, and turn your palms towards each other in a mirror image of Step 1. Repeat the sequence several times and note how it becomes more fluid.

# 26 mind-sharpening yoga

Yoga is one of the best ways to keep the joints and muscles flexible. It can relieve problems such as stress and anxiety, depression, back pain, asthma and insomnia – all of which can sap your energy.

**the tree pose**

To do this classical asana (yoga pose), stand with your feet hip–width apart, toes evenly spread. Allow your right leg to float up, bent at the knee. Take hold of your right foot and position the sole against the inner thigh of your standing leg, with the bent knee out to the side. If you cannot achieve this, place the sole where it is comfortable on the inside of the straight leg. Realign your pelvis, tucking your tailbone under, and softly fix your gaze on a point in front of you to help you balance. When you feel steady, raise your arms like the branches of a tree, breathing in. Hold the position for several breaths, and bring leg and arms down on an out-breath. Repeat with the opposite leg.

When you have worked both sides, stand with knees bent and drop the trunk forward and down, arms and head hanging loosely. This is excellent for neck exercises, as the weight of the head helps to extend the cervical spine. Move your head up gently, also breathing gently to loosen any tension. Uncurl your spine slowly and bring your chin up last, then rest.

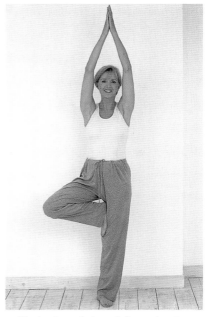

▲ *The best way to learn is from a teacher, but this exercise may be tried safely at home.*

Balancing poses sharpen the mind as well as exercising a lot of "inner" muscles. If balance is a problem, lean against a wall and experiment with the position of the bent leg. Your mental outlook should improve, too.

# 27 uplifting oils

Aromatherapy treatments can be an effective means of restoring vitality and helping body and soul to recuperate after illness; citrus oils are very good at lifting moods and improving energy levels.

### invigorating bath

Try this bath for a strong boost to the system, either in the morning or as a special afternoon reviving session.

4 drops of bergamot oil
2 drops of neroli oil
several drops of almond
    or wheatgerm oil

Fill the bathtub with warm water, then swirl essential oil drops in the bath just before getting in, so that their potency is at its height. Settle into the water and breathe in the stimulating scent.

### sensual oil burner

Another way to benefit from the healing power of essential oils is to use an oil burner. Add 1 or 2 drops of bergamot oil and/or 1 of neroli to the top of an essential oil burner and light the candle. The scent will pervade the atmosphere, providing you with a steady dose of the oils' uplifting substances. Experiment with the many oils available.

▾ *The pungent scent of essential oils can permeate a room with a burst of powerful energy. Try using on a foggy winter's day.*

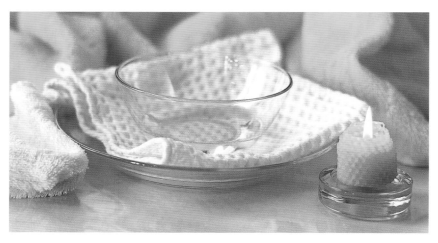

Imagine beginning your day by soaking in a refreshing bath filled with exotic flowers and spices.

Transport yourself to the midst of a pine forest, an oriental spice market or a citrus orange grove with just a few drops of essential oil.

# 29 invigorating bath oil

Herbal baths can be used for therapeutic purposes to raise energy levels and stimulate the senses. Simply scatter sprigs of herbs in the bath water or use their concentrated oil essences.

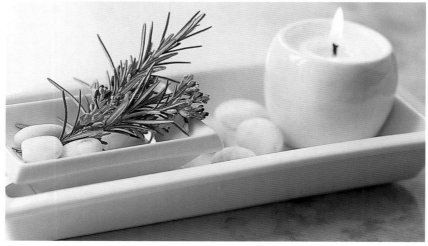

For a simple bath using essential oils, first draw the water and then measure out 5 drops. The oils form a thin film on the surface, and this, aided by the warmth of the water, will be partly absorbed by the skin.

**milk & honey**
**bath oil with rosemary**
The milk in this bath will leave your skin silky smooth.
2 eggs
45ml/3 tbsp rosemary oil
10ml/2 tsp honey

▲ *The heady scent of rosemary provides an immediate physical and psychological uplift.*

10ml/2 tsp baby or other
   mild shampoo
15ml/1 tbsp vodka
150ml/¼ pint/⅔ cup milk

Beat the eggs and oil together, then add the other ingredients and mix thoroughly. Pour into a clean glass bottle. Add 30-45ml/2-3 tbsp to the bath and keep the remainder chilled until ready for further use.

# 30 instant revitalizing massage

At any time of the day, energy levels can flag: after a meeting, when taking the children to school or out shopping. You can give yourself a quick "wake-up call" by doing this effective self-massage routine.

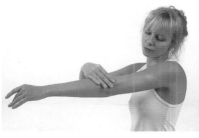

**1** First, knead the arms, working rapidly from wrist to shoulder and back again with a firm squeezing movement. Next, rub swiftly upwards on the outside arm to stimulate circulation.

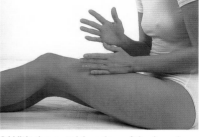

**3** With the outside edge of the hands, lightly hack on the front of each thigh, using a rapid motion. Do not karate-chop the thighs – the hands should spring up from the muscles.

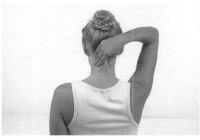

**2** With the fingers and thumb of one hand, firmly squeeze your neck muscles using a gentle circular motion. Slowly work up the neck and then back down again. Continue the exercise until you feel the muscles have loosened.

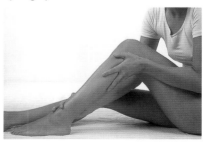

**4** Now rub the calves vigorously to loosen them and get the blood flowing. It is best to do this with the knees bent. Work from the ankle to the knee, using alternating hands. Finally, stand up and shake your entire body, to let go of any stiffness and tensions.

# 31 re-balancing reflexology

Reflexology attempts to address imbalances in the body by applying pressure to corresponding points on the feet. The therapy encourages the healing and restoration of the body's equilibrium.

## energy level enhancer

These simple reflexology exercises will help to stimulate the flow of energy through particular areas. Each section marked on the foot represents a different part of the body. Try the treatments on your own feet, or get a friend to help. Rest for a half hour after the treatment; your organs need time to readjust after stimulation.

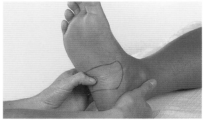

**3** Work the small intestines to aid the uptake of nutrients.

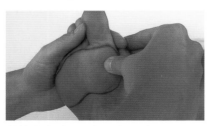

**1** Work the lungs in order to improve your breathing.

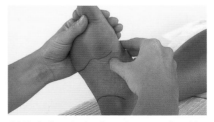

**4** Work the whole digestive area: food is turned into energy during digestion.

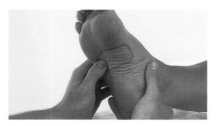

**2** Work the liver; many of its functions are crucial to your health and stamina.

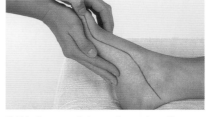

**5** Work up and down the spine, the central column of your energy flow.

# 32 restorative flowers

Developed by Dr Edward Bach in the early 20th century, Bach flower remedies work on the premise that flower essences can enhance energy levels by restoring positive feelings and emotions.

Available from good-quality health food shops, Bach flower essences are sold separately. You can either ask your health practitioner to create tailor-made treatments for you, or try the following combinations:

### exhaustion mix
Elm, Gorse, Hornbeam, Mustard, Oak, Olive, Walnut and Rose. This mix is useful as a pick-me-up after prolonged periods of work; it is also useful when responsibilities place a drain on the system.

### confidence mix
Centaury, Chestnut Bud, Gentian, Larch, Pine, Sweet Chestnut, Walnut and Wild Rose. Helps to build inner confidence and constancy.

### work stress mix
Gentian, Hornbeam, Impatiens, Mustard, Olive, Rock Water, Vervain, Walnut and White Chestnut. This mixture refreshes and restores interest when you are under stress at work. The Emergency Essence mix is also useful during stressful or anxious situations of any variety.

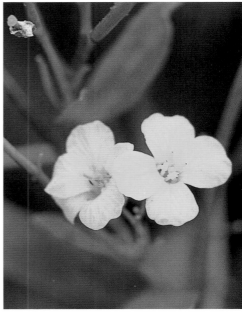

▲ By taking Bach remedies, you may find relief from stress and build up your inner resources, thereby energizing body and soul.

### study and intuition mix
Cerato, Chestnut Bud, Clematis, Impatiens, Rock Water, Scleranthus, White Chestnut and Wild Oat. Helps with concentration during work and study, and boosts enthusiasm.

# 33 colour stimulants

Different colours can be used to stimulate and revive the senses, giving body and mind a real lift. Choose warm, vibrant shades for clothes, food and furnishings as part of your energizing strategy.

## exhilarating wardrobe

For a reviving colour hit, choose clothes of red, orange and yellow hues, which are hot and stimulating. Red gives you extra energy and heals lethargy and tiredness, while orange is said to create optimism and change, at the same time acting to heal grief and disappointment. To encourage more laughter, joy and fun in your life, and to keep depression at bay, opt for yellow clothes and accessories. Warm colours make your skin glow and work to attract other people, making you feel more vibrant and sociable.

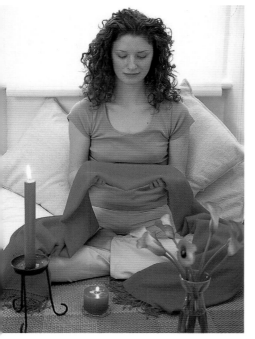

▲ *Stimulating high-energy colours, such as red, orange and yellow, can help activate your passion for life.*

## happy interiors

Colour in the home or workplace can have a big impact on productivity. Paint the kitchen a glowing yellow to add cheer and inspire your cooking experience. Solid red or orange walls in a room can be overpowering, but you can easily splash accents of these hues in a room to increase mental alacrity. Spring green shades also have a livening effect.

## mood foods

If you want to increase your zest for life, choose "passionate" foods – red strawberries and cherries, orange carrots and pumpkins, yellow peppers and squashes. Organic foods, grown without additives, are best.

# 34 energizing crystals

When the body is in a state of imbalance, a lack of energy is often felt. Correcting the balance using crystal techniques may help to restore and augment your physical stamina.

Red, orange and yellow crystals have the effect of promoting an increase in energy. Bright, strong colours – such as a deep-red garnet, golden amber or topaz – are very dynamic and stimulating. The more earthy tones of tiger's eye, citrine and jasper tend to foster an increase in practical motivation, so these are good to use when you need an energy boost for specific chores or projects.

You may find some of the stones too energizing at certain times. For example, golden citrine quartz is a wonderful substitute for the sun's warm energy – but on a hot summer's day, you might find it uncomfortable. Experiment with the stones, and soon you will know what each can do, and which is best for a particular situation.

## QUICK FIX
To provide a quick burst of energy, recline comfortably and hold one clear quartz crystal – pointed upwards – in each hand. Place a large citrine at the solar plexus. Remain in position until you feel the stone's energy has "recharged" you.

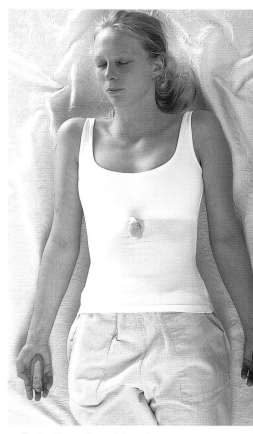

▲ *During times of special need, you can give yourself an extra boost by using stones that directly stimulate vitality.*

# 35 arousing bath oils

Effective treatments for dry skin, bath blends with uplifting essential oils can also have a beneficial influence on mood and health. The base oils in this recipe – almond and wheatgerm – are very gentle.

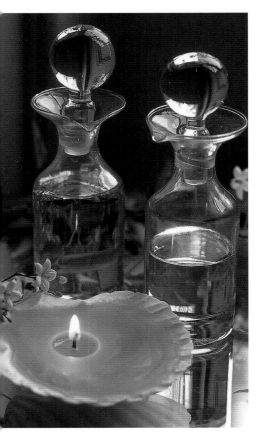

**grapefruit and coriander bath oil**
The combination of grapefruit and coriander has a wonderfully refreshing and arousing effect on the system, and the base oils soothe and calm flaky, dry skin. This blend is a potent reviver for times when you are recovering from a cold or flu.

100ml/3½fl oz/scant ½ cup almond oil
20ml/4 tsp wheatgerm oil
30 drops grapefruit essential oil
30 drops coriander essential oil
opaque glass bottle

Mix all of the ingredients in the bottle and shake well. Pour about 1 tbsp into the bath just prior to getting in and swirl to disperse. This recipe makes about 120ml/4fl oz/scant ½ cup.

> **CAUTION**
> When using citrus oils such as grapefruit, orange and lemon for the first time, try a small amount – the acids in citrus can sometimes irritate very sensitive skin. Always keep oils away from the eyes.

▲ *Bath blends are simple to make at home and they are chemical-free – so you know exactly what you are putting on your skin.*

# 36 reviving rose bath salts

Bath blends that contain a mixture of salts and aromatic flowers or herbs have long been used to treat a variety of complaints. Although many salts can be used, this blend uses simple sea salt.

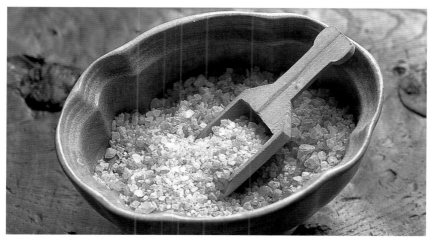

**rose bath salts**
10g/¼oz dried rose petals
mortar and pestle or electric
    coffee grinder
500g/1¼lb coarse sea salt
10 drops rose geranium essential oil
5 drops lavender essential oil
5 drops bergamot essential oil
decorative 500g/1¼lb glass jar,
    with close-fitting lid

Grind all but a handful of the rose petals (left whole for decoration). Mix the ground petals into the salt. Add the essential oils; stir thoroughly.

▲ Soak in a bath of aromatic rose bath salts to scent the skin and lift the spirits.

Spoon into the jar, adding a layer of whole rose petals halfway up. Place the lid on firmly and store in a cool, dry place. Makes about 500g/1¼lb.

**how to use bath salts**
Add 2 heaped tablespoons to running water in a medium-hot bath – if the water is too hot, the salt may elevate your heart rate and irritate your skin. Get in the tub and immerse yourself for a maximum of 15 minutes.

# 37 ginger body scrub

With its invigorating aroma and chemical action, ginger stimulates circulation, making it an excellent ingredient for an energizing body scrub. Clay and honey clean the skin by drawing out impurities.

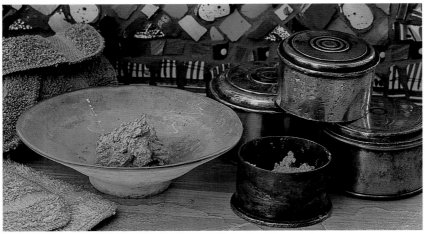

**ginger and honey scrub**
2 small bowls
20ml/4 tsp kaolin
10ml/2 tsp green clay
15ml/1 tbsp ground almonds
15ml/1 tbsp clear honey
30ml/2 tbsp warm water
15ml/1 tbsp orange flower water
3 drops ginger essential oil
small spoon
glass storage jar

*▲ Rejuvenate your skin with a fresh scrub.*

In one bowl, place the kaolin, green clay and ground almonds. In the other, dissolve the honey in the water, and then add the orange flower water and essential oil. Slowly pour the honey, water, orange flower and oil mixture into the kaolin, clay and ground almond mixture. Blend the mixture using the spoon. To use, massage into the skin in a circular motion, adding a little water if necessary. Rinse off with warm water. It is best to use all the scrub in one treatment, but you can store the remainder in a glass jar in the refrigerator for up to 4 weeks.

# 38 tansy skin freshener

Tansy leaves have a strong, singular scent, and the plant is easy to grow. Pick fresh leaves for this invigorating skin tonic, and use it in the morning to give your skin a garden-fresh start to the day.

In ancient Greece, tansy was said to have been given to Ganymede to make him immortal. The herbalist Culpeper claimed it was a cure for diseases of the skin. Today, tansy's known tonic and stimulant qualities make it an ideal skin freshener.

**tansy freshener**
1 large handful of tansy leaves
150ml/¼ pint/⅔ cup water
150ml/¼ pint/⅔ cup milk
pan
strainer
jar

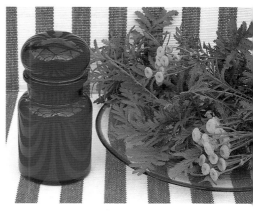

▲ *Tansy tonic will invigorate your skin first thing in the morning.*

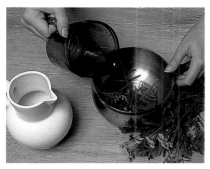

**1** Place all the ingredients in a small pan and bring to the boil. Simmer for 15 minutes, then remove from the heat and allow to cool.

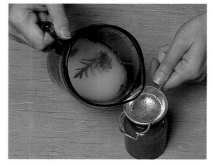

**2** Strain the liquid into a glass jar. Store the tonic in the refrigerator and apply cold to the skin for a refreshing jolt of energy.

# 39

## lemon verbena
## hair rinse

This rinse stimulates the pores and circulation of the scalp – and it bestows a wonderful, invigorating fragrance upon your hair. Use the fresh leaves of the lemon verbena plant for this recipe.

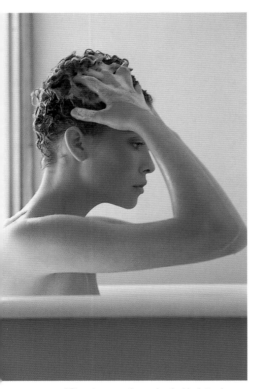

**lemon verbena rinse**
250ml/8fl oz/1 cup boiling water
1 handful of lemon verbena leaves
bowl
jug (pitcher)
strainer

Place the lemon verbena leaves in a bowl and pour the boiling water over. Set aside to infuse for at least one hour. Strain the liquid and discard the leaves. After normal washing and conditioning, pour the rinse over your hair, covering the strands and scalp. Dry and style as usual.

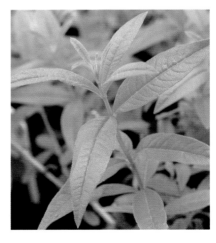

▲ *After shampooing, a herbal hair tonic can enhance circulation of the scalp, leaving it feeling tingling and refreshed.*

▶ *Lemon verbena has a multitude of uses and is easily grown in the garden.*

# 40   mint foot treatments

Soaking tired feet at the end of the day will revitalize your whole body. Follow a foot bath with a mint rub to smooth and soften aching feet before going to bed, preparing them for the next day.

You can use mint, peppermint or spearmint leaves and essential oil for these soothing treatments; they all contain cooling menthol. Choose your favourite.

**mint foot bath**
12 sprigs fresh mint
blender or food processor
120ml/4fl oz/½ cup cold water
large bowl
2.2 litres/4 pints/9 cups boiling water

Place the mint in a food processor and add the cold water. Process to a green purée. Pour the purée into a large bowl and add the boiling water. Let cool to just a bearable temperature, then soak both feet at once, until the water is no longer comforting.

**mint foot massage oil**
15ml/1 tbsp almond oil
1 drop mint essential oil

After bathing in the foot bath, gently dry your feet with a soft towel. Mix the almond oil and the mint essential oil together, and then rub thoroughly into both feet.

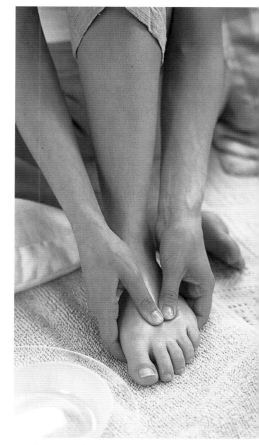

▲ *Mint opens the pores and cleanses the skin, leaving it cool and pleasantly tingling.*

Step into a
cold shower to provide
a gentle shock to a
sluggish system. You will feel
instantly refreshed
and wide awake.

# 42 go for a brisk walk

Walking is one of the simplest and most effective forms of exercise. It is a means of accelerating your physical energy levels and consequently raising your spirits – and it is enjoyable.

You can walk almost anywhere, and by going outside, you immediately change your environment to give you a new angle on your situation. Of course, walking provides many physiological benefits: it boosts your heart rate and respiration, speeds up your metabolism, tones your muscles and brings more oxygen to your bloodstream. It also causes the body to produce endorphins – the "feel good" hormones – which lift your mood and strengthen your immune system, helping to keep illness at bay.

**meditation on the go**

Walking can be a form of meditation, too. When you're feeling fed up or annoyed, try taking a gentle stroll around the block. As you walk along, it is likely that your problems will begin to feel less acute. It is almost as though the physical steps are mental steps that bring you closer to understanding difficult situations or overcoming obstacles.

▶ *Just taking a 10-15 minute walk can help you put any problems in perspective, and aid you in coming up with new solutions.*

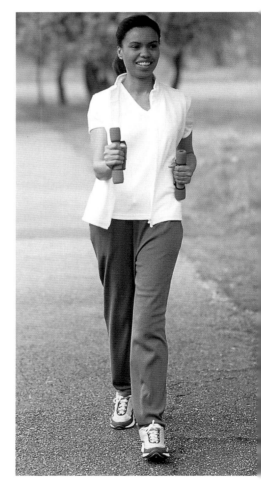

# 43

## practise deep breathing

The power of proper breathing should not be underestimated – it oxygenates the blood, aiding thought processes and boosting physical energy. This simple technique can be carried out anywhere.

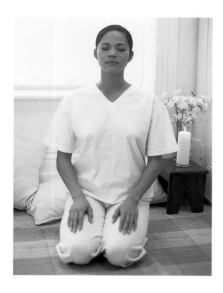

◂ *With regular practice, deep breathing can reduce stress on your nervous system.*

Many people do not breathe properly, taking shallow or quick gulps of air. By breathing from the diaphragm, you will bring oxygen all the way to the bottom of your lungs. This will improve your circulation, enhancing the body's systems and energy levels.

### exercise and visualize

When practising deep breathing, there are many ways of concentrating the mind in order to heighten your physical stamina and mood, and to help quell the negative inner "voice" that can drain your reserves and dampen your spirits.

**1** Start by counting your breaths, evenly, from one to ten.

**2** Note the physical changes at the nostrils and the abdomen, as your breath moves in and out.

**3** Notice the inner stillness as you change from exhalation to inhalation, from inhalation to exhalation. Now imagine drawing new energy into your lungs with each breath.

**4** Close your eyes and conjure up an image that evokes a feeling of wholeness, joy and serenity. This could be a beautiful, natural scene with mountains or a valley, the undulating waves of the ocean, the sun's bright rays or a child you are fond of. Breathe in this complete image, until you feel its fresh, positive energy permeating throughout your entire body and mind.

**5** Open your eyes and enjoy your feelings of renewed vigour.

# 44

# inhale a scent

The sense of smell is the most primal of the five physical senses, and – although often played down in modern societies – it can be stimulated in many ways to evoke positive, invigorating feelings.

### surround yourself with flowers

When feeling tired or low, give your mood an instant lift by buying a bunch of bright, luscious-scented flowers and placing them in a vase in your home or office. Choose from delicate freesias, roses and strong-scented star lilies; or daffodils, narcissi and hyacinths – which can be grown in pots indoors, in winter and spring.

### evocative essential oils

Aromatherapy advocates using oil burners to disperse essentials oils in a room. Place a few drops in the burner and light the candle beneath. Mints such as peppermint and spearmint are very stimulating, as are orange, geranium and ylang ylang. You can experiment with myriad different combinations of your favourite oils. Another way to experience oils is to place a few drops in a warm bath.

### baking boost

The smell of baking bread or biscuits (cookies) can be a real mood booster – vanilla in particular triggers happy memories of childhood for many people. Choose a nutritious wholemeal

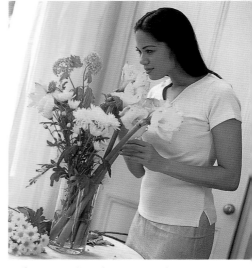

▲ *Scent can trigger happy memories.*

bread or biscuit recipe, and set to work – delicious aromas will soon waft through your house, putting a smile on your face.

### refreshing air

Simply open a window to experience all the smells of grass, trees, blossoms, soil and rain outside. Even in winter, it can be very stimulating to let in the fresh air for just a few minutes.

# 45

## eat a high-protein lunch

Do you often experience a mid-afternoon slump after eating a proper lunch? The cause may be foods that are high in fast-burning carbohydrates, leaving you with an energy deficit by around 3:00pm.

Many people's lives are too active to stop for a siesta during the afternoon; therefore, planning a lunch that provides sustaining energy through a busy working day is essential. Try a meal that includes high-protein chicken or tuna. Vegetarians may want to choose eggs, hummus or Quorn (mico-protein meat substitute), all of which are processed by the digestive system at a slower rate than carbohydrates and will provide energy for a longer period of time.

▼ By choosing high-protein fish, you will feed your body with slower-burning fuel.

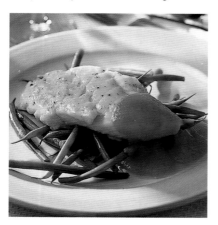

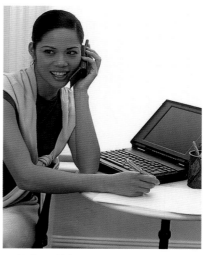

▲ Eating a high-protein lunch will help to sustain you throughout the afternoon.

### protein snacking

When you do experience mid-afternoon hunger pangs, it's best not to reach for the biscuits (cookies) and chocolate – you'll be back in the same boat as before. These snacks are high in sugars that quickly disturb glucose levels, giving your body a rapid sugar rush, but leaving you feeling fatigued an hour later. Instead, grab a handful of nuts, or a rye cracker with cheese.

# 46 have a laugh

It has often been said that laughter is the best medicine. Research has confirmed this maxim: laughter raises endorphin levels, alleviating stress and allowing body and mind to work energetically.

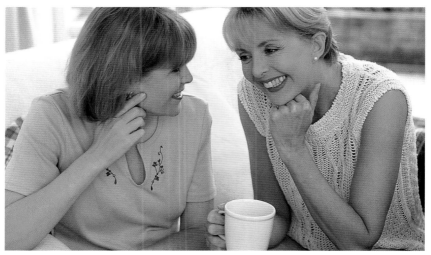

**chuckle your way through the day**
• Share a joke with a close friend or a group of friends, via talking, text messaging or email.
• Write down any funny thoughts that you may have and turn them into little stories. If you're good at drawing, make cartoons of the characters with captions.
• Try and see the silly side of serious or stressful situations: the best-adjusted people can laugh at most things, from disasters to death.
• Don't be afraid to laugh at yourself

▲ *People who laugh a lot are healthier overall. Fun is a very important aspect of life that should never be overlooked.*

and your own foibles. Everyone makes mistakes, and at least they can be enjoyed and rate as entertainment value in retrospect.

**when feeling low key...**
• Plan a night out at a comedy club with a group of friends.
• Watch videos of your favourite film or comedy series.

# get up & dance

A highly aerobic activity, dancing wakes up the system in no uncertain terms – and it makes you feel great. Cares and worries quickly melt away after the first few minutes of a good boogie.

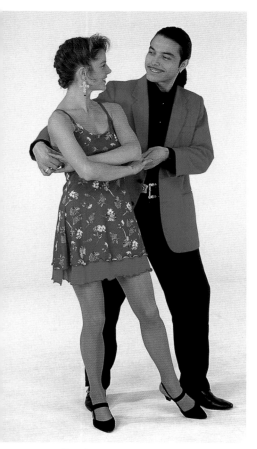

▲ *Dancing burns stress-related adrenaline and leaves you feeling wonderfully energized.*

Dancing has developed in all world cultures as a means of celebrating life. It is one of the most enjoyable ways to express yourself and to exercise. Many gyms offer classes in various styles: for example, salsa, samba, ceroc, jazz and ballroom. You may want to choose a highly vigorous dance form, such as rock 'n' roll; or perhaps choose one that is lower key, such as free-form or line dancing.

Some complex routines – such as those found in Indian and Indonesian classical forms – will keep your mind occupied with their intricate moves, and you will experience a real sense of accomplishment when you learn each sequence. Egyptian belly dancing is good for toning the midriff.

### solo practice

Much enjoyment can be had by dancing with others, but you can also simply turn on your favourite up-tempo CD and dance by yourself, for a private workout guaranteed to enliven body and soul. If you are shy about dancing in public, this is the perfect prelude to going to a club with friends or signing up for a dance class.

# 48 think positively

Instead of concentrating on a daily catalogue of mishaps and frustrations or your own lack of luck, you can invigorate your life experience by looking on the bright side of everyday situations.

The power of positive thinking is so strong that it will help you overcome obstacles and create solutions to pressing problems. It will enable you to enjoy what you think and do, giving you new hope and energy.

**life on the bright side**
Negativity only serves to sap your inner resources. For example, if your car doesn't start in the morning and needs an all-day repair, it is easy to think your day is ruined. But looking on the positive side of the situation, you might just shrug your shoulders and say, "Oh well... this gives me a chance to work on a project at home today. I've been needing some time to myself..." In this way, you are not using up precious energy by allowing yourself to be ruled by anger and frustration – you are actually creating positive energy by seeing a challenge as an opportunity to do something enjoyable and rewarding.

Positive thinking can be applied to almost any scenario, enhancing your feelings of self-confidence and perhaps leading you to explore possibilities hitherto hidden.

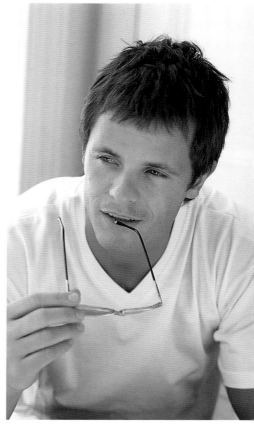

▲ *It is a good idea to start the day by "counting your blessings" – review all the good things you have, and go on from there.*

# 49 clear your mind

Feeling overwhelmed or bogged down with too much to do can lead to low energy levels at best, depression at worst. Clearing your mind of "excess baggage" can do wonders to improve your mood.

## have a clear out

Sometimes a clear out of your physical environment can work wonders for your frame of mind. Set aside an evening to sort through old or unwanted clothes and get rid of them, giving them to friends or a charity shop. You will not only make way for new clothes, you will give yourself space for exciting new thoughts and feelings as well. In a similar way, you can clear a room or work space, creating more physical space and therefore more "head" or mental space in which to generate stimulating new ideas and solutions.

## finishing projects

You may have so many tasks to complete in the course of a day, that your "to do" list becomes highly unmanageable. It is tempting to start something, then move on to the next "tick" in a panic. This will only frustrate and sap your energy, leaving you with a sense that nothing is ever completed. Try to create a reasonable list of tasks that you know you can accomplish, and do one thing at a time. Your list will magically diminish.

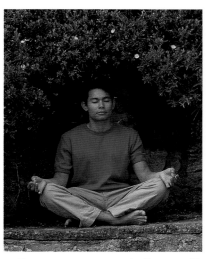

▲ *Use your energy economically – spend it on people and things that really matter.*

## meditation time

Practising meditation is a pleasant way to energize, one in which you allow precious time and space for yourself. Meditation can help you to clear your mind of unwanted thoughts and feelings – perhaps some that have been holding you back for a long time. It can help you come to terms with situations and people over which you have no control.

# 50

## have a good night's sleep

The value of sleep is too often underrated. To maintain our energy levels for the often hectic round of daily work, domestic and even leisure activities, a good night's sleep is essential.

Although we spend a third of our lives asleep, the importance of sleep is still something of a mystery. The body expends almost as much energy asleep as it does awake, and it is known that sleep is important for growth, learning and memory. Anyone who has suffered from insomnia will know that a lack of sleep causes irritability and poor concentration; if prolonged for greater periods, it can even cause ill health and hallucinations. A good night's sleep can be conducive to creativity – not only for artistic pursuits, but for the handling of the myriad daily tasks and challenges.

### inspiring dreams

Many psychologists believe that dreams provide an important key to a person's mental and emotional health. It is thought that we work through problems and feelings when we dream, leaving us to wake with a fresh perspective. Dreams can also provide inspiration and insights, shedding light on intuitive knowledge and talents – and they can be highly enjoyable as a personal entertainment system, tuned in to our own "channel".

### practical sleep aids

• Get plenty of exercise during the day, preferably out in the fresh air.
• Restrict coffee and tea to three cups a day; refrain from caffeine after 6pm.
• Take a warm – not hot – bath, about an hour before going to bed.
• Drink a cup of herbal tea or a hot, milky drink to soothe you to sleep.

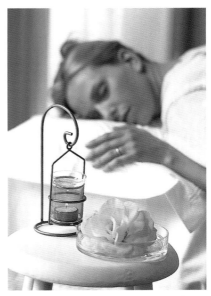

▲ Create a peaceful bedroom atmosphere with soft lighting and soothing scents.

# index

aerobic exercise, 8, 32
anaerobic exercise, 8, 33
antioxidants, 7, 12, 13, 16
aromatherapy, 8, 38–40, 55

Bach flower remedies, 43
backwards bend, 34
baking, 55
balancing poses, 37
banana and strawberry
    smoothie, 31
baths, 38–40, 46–7, 51
beans, 18
beef, 22
berry yogurt shake, 30
body scrub, ginger and
    honey, 48
bread, garlic, 25
breathing, 54
burners, oil, 38, 55

cereals, 17
citrus shake, 30
clutter, 60
colour: colour healing,
    8, 44
  crystal healing, 8, 45

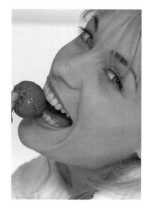

cranberry and apple juice,
    27
crystal healing, 8, 45

dancing, 58
dreams, 61
drinks, 26–31

eggs, 20
endorphins, 8, 53, 57
exercise, 7–8, 32–7, 53, 58

fats, 19, 23

feet: mint foot bath, 51
  mint foot massage oil, 51
  reflexology, 42
fibre, 17
fish, 19
fish posture, 34
flowers: flower remedies, 43
  scent, 55
  tisanes, 29
food, 7, 16–25
  colour healing, 44
  high-protein lunch, 56
fruit, 12, 16
  juices, 27
  shakes, 30
  smoothies, 31

garlic, 25
ginger and honey body
    scrub, 48
grains, 17
grapefruit and coriander
    bath oil, 46

hair rinse, lemon verbena, 50
healing: colour healing,
    8, 44
  crystal healing, 8, 45
herbs: baths, 40
  herbal teas, 28

immune system, 15
iron, 15, 22

juices, 27

laughter, 57

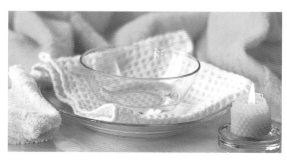

# index

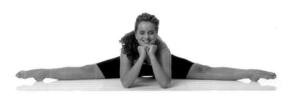
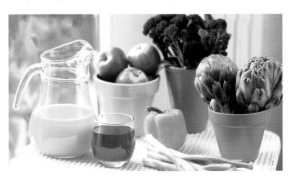

This edition is published by Lorenz Books,
an imprint of Anness Publishing Ltd,
Blaby Road, Wigston, Leicestershire LE18 4SE; info@anness.com

www.lorenzbooks.com;
www.annesspublishing.com

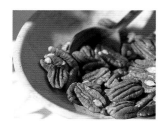

If you like the images in this book and would like to investigate using them for
publishing, promotions or advertising, please visit our website
www.practicalpictures.com for more information.

A CIP catalogue record for this book is available from the British Library.

Publisher: Joanna Lorenz
Managing editor: Helen Sudell
Editor: Melanie Halton
Designer: Carlton Hibbert
Photography: Simon Bottomley, Martin Brigdale, Nick Cole, John Freeman,
Michelle Garrett, Christine Hanscomb, Amanda Heywood, Janine Hosegood, Andrea
Jones, Don Last, Liz McAulay, Steve Moss, Thomas Odulate, Anthony Pickhaver, Fiona
Pragoff, Craig Robertson and Simon Smith
Production manager: Steve Lang
Indexer: Hilary Bird

**Publisher's note:**
The reader should not regard the recommendations, ideas and techniques expressed and
described in this book as substitutes for the advice of a qualified medical practitioner or
other qualified professional. Any use to which the recommendations, ideas and
techniques are put is at the reader's sole discretion and risk.

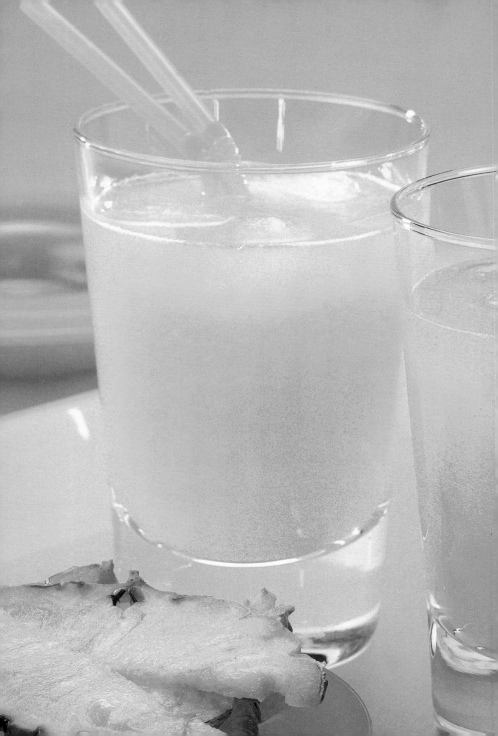